HELPFUL TIPS
for
TRACHEOSTOMY CARE

Coretta Johnson

Copyright © 2013 by Coretta Johnson. 120987-JOHN

ISBN: Softcover   978-1-4797-2499-4
        Hardcover   978-1-4797-2500-7
        Ebook   978-1-4797-2501-4

All rights reserved. No part of this book may be reproduced or transmitted in any form or by any means, electronic or mechanical, including photocopying, recording, or by any information storage and retrieval system, without permission in writing from the copyright owner.

Rev. Date:02/28/2013

To order additional copies of this book, contact:
Xlibris Corporation
1-888-795-4274
www.Xlibris.com
Orders@Xlibris.com

Table of Contents

Acknowledgment 2
CHAPTER 1:   Hospital Stay.. 4
    The NICU 4
    Transferred To The PICU 8
    I Can See Your Face 9
CHAPTER 2:   Moving to Rehabilitation Hospital... 11
    Road Trip To Rehab 11
    Coping With Relocating To Rehab 11
CHAPTER 3:   Going Home 17
    Finally Going Home 16
    Choosing The Right Nurses... 19
    Choosing The Right Therapist... 21
CHAPTER 4:   Tracheotomy Care 26
    Trach Time 26
    Preparing Supplies For Trach Maintenance Or Trach Tube Change................ 28
    Suctioning 30
    Infection Control 32
    Six Important House Rules To Reduce Infection.. 32
CHAPTER 5:   Possible Side Effects of Tracheotomy 34
    Possible Side Effects Of Having Tracheotomy 34
    Presurgery Tips 36
    Some Extra Tips That Worked For Me.. 37
Sweet Reunion Pictures 40
Index 42

Acknowledgment

Thank you God! For giving me the strength to get through the most difficult five years of my life, and for choosing my mother, Zelina Elsa Lloyd (a.k.a Grandma Nina), to care for me in this world. Thank you for giving up your life to help me through the most difficult time in my life. Thank you for giving me the push to follow my dreams and never give up. Thank you for telling me when I am wrong, but most importantly, thank you for being the best mother one could ever ask for.

To my husband, Theophilus Johnson, thank you for motivating me because of your positive words, I push myself to keep going. I cannot thank you enough.

To my wonderful siblings, Beverley Prince, Patricia Lloyd-Jackson and Philip Lloyd, thank you for always having my back and for listening to me when I was down. Philip, extra thanks for all the nights you stayed up with me when I was sick.

To my nieces and nephew, thanks for the support, love you bunches.

To Aunt Margaret, thanks for loving me no matter what and for always being there when I needed you most.

To my mother-in-law, Gloria Johnson, thanks for all your continuing support.

To my sisters-in-law, Joy Lloyd and Andrea Wilcock, thank you for all your support, you will always hold a special place in my heart; may God continue to bless both of you with good health especially you, WA.

To my most loyal friends, Lisa, Gail, Wendy, and Caren, thanks for being my therapist or my shoulder to cry on. Each of you hold a special place in my heart, and are all very dear to me, you all have special qualities that are priceless.

To Father Gunthorpes, thank you for keeping us in your prayers; thank you for listening when I needed it most.

Special thanks to my team of nurses, Trinity, Theresa (God bless her soul) and Annette, thank you for putting up with me, and for understanding that we work as a team. I could not have cared for Thea without your help. Trinity, thanks for always going the extra mile.

Special thanks to Dr. Cao and Dr. R Ward, thank you for always listening, returning every phone call and for working with me for the best interest of my child. I wish every parent has doctors like you.

To everyone who supported me, you know who you are; I could not thank you enough, and I am blessed to have you in my life.

CHAPTER 1

Hospital Stay

THE NICU

My daughter (Thea) was born prematurely at twenty seven weeks; her birth weight was two pounds and two ounces. She was able to breathe on her own for about two weeks, at which time I noticed she was breathing too fast for a baby (as if she was running a marathon). It was my first clue that she was in trouble. I notified the doctors of my concerns, she was diagnosed with *chronic lung disease*—her lungs were not fully developed. Due to her prematurity and not breathing on her own, her lungs became more damaged and very brittle with elasticity. She began to have difficulty breathing on her own (respiratory distress) which resulted in her being intubated.

Intubation is a medical procedure in which a tube is placed into the windpipe (trachea) through the mouth or the nose. In Thea's case, it was through her mouth. A large tube was placed above her head and a mechanical ventilator was attached to the tube to give her breaths

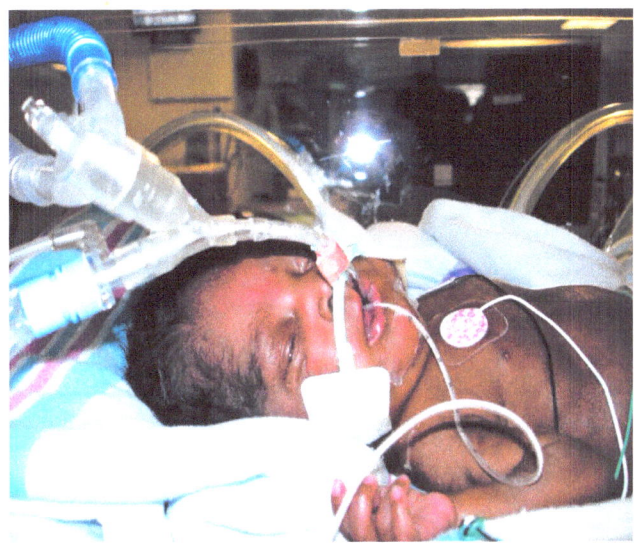

Photograph 1. Ventilator attached to tube to give her breaths

For several weeks, she was intubated on two other machines: Oscillator and Diffusive Volumetric Respirator (DVR). The Oscillator is a machine that helps a baby to breathe. The machine delivers short, low-volume breaths per minute, which causes a baby's chest to jiggle instead of rise and fall as normally would. The difference between the ventilator and the Oscillator is that the ventilator gives breaths but the oscillator gives breaths and shakes. In some cases, the child can get used to the shaking motion of the Oscillator (it can be very comforting and soothing), which is what occurred with Thea. The Oscillator comforted her so the doctors kept her on the machine longer than they had initially planned. After several attempts to remove her were unsuccessful due to her attachment, she had to be gradually taken off the machine.

Thea's condition took a turn for the worse after she was taken off of the Oscillator. I received the phone call that every parent with a premature child in the NICU dreads; the call that she might not make it. I rushed to the hospital as fast as I could with my mother on my heel. When I got there, I noticed the doctors and respiratory therapists around her cubicle, and the worst feeling in the world hit me. The machines were bleeping, her numbers (O2) were between zero and fifty —there was nothing else they could do. I just wanted to hold her so I asked the doctor if I could, and she said yes; but then it hit me that when a child is on an Oscillator, you can't hold them. I asked the doctor if it is a bad sign that I am allowed to hold her and she said yes. I took Thea in my arms and kissed her. Her numbers or stats improved between 95 and 100. We were all shocked at her immediate improvement and I asked them to put her back. She just wanted to be hugged and held.

After Thea's miraculous improvement, I was willing to try anything as she was willing to fight; I had to help her. I begged them to do whatever they had to do to help her. The head of the respiratory department suggested the use of a *Diffusive Volumetric Respirator* (DVR), a life support system that delivers a unique form of ventilation which expands the lungs. I told them I would sign whatever they wanted me to sign because it was better than doing nothing, and at least I knew I tried. This type of machine had not been used in any other hospital in the tri-state area. This hospital was the only hospital with this machine, which made her the first baby to use this machine. This was a challenge because the machine was new, and the respiratory therapist was not familiar with it, but with their determination, round-the-clock monitoring, and prayers, I am happy to say it saved her life.

Thea stayed on the DVR for about one week and she was then transferred to *Continuous Positive Airway Pressure* (CPAP). CPAP delivers oxygen to her body using a small amount of pressure through a little tube that fits into the nostrils (shown in photograph 2 below). This process helps to keep the air sacs in the lungs opened.

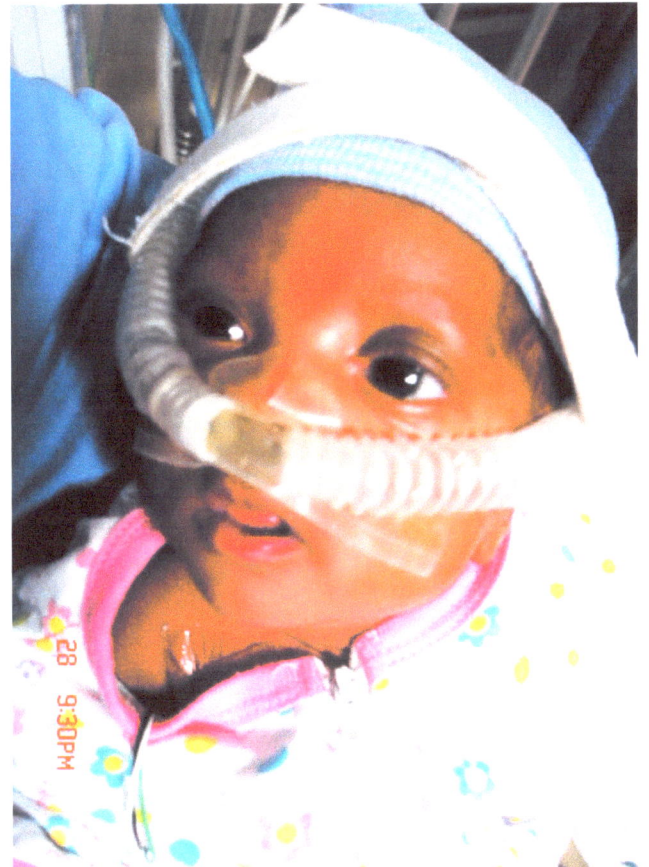

Photograph 2. Continuous Positive Airway Pressure (CPAP)

After several attempts to remove the tube for her to breathe on her own were unsuccessful (she was almost four moths old by this time), I wondered what the next step would be to help her. It was obvious that they had done all they could for her at this point in the NICU.

The NICU doctors thought a fresh team of doctors might be the best course of action for her at this point, and she was transferred to the Pediatric Intensive Care Unit (PICU) for further care.

At first I thought the doctors in the NICU were giving up on her, and as a parent, I felt helpless. Her condition was not getting any better. The doctors kept telling me her lungs were too brittle, stiff and weak for her to breathe on her own. I looked at my child; I would give her my lung, if that was an option.

TRANSFERRED TO THE PICU

The decision to transfer her to PICU was the best decision they ever made. There is an additional up side to moving to PICU unit, you can stay with your child around the clock which was easier for me and my family. At the end of the first week, Thea was greeted by a new set of doctors which included a pediatric doctor, respiratory therapist, pulmonologists, otorhinolaryngologist and nurses to assist with her condition.

She was reevaluated and the team of doctors decided the best course of action for her condition was a *tracheotomy*. This procedure would relieve some of the pressure on her lungs and give the lungs time to grow and heal. I was willing to try anything at this point as long as she was able to breathe. I had less than forty eight hours to learn everything I could about tracheotomy which can be overwhelming on any parent. I asked one of the nurses to break it down as simple as possible. She explained to me all the advantages and disadvantages of having a trach.

The tracheotomy was performed when Thea was five months old (shown in the photograph 3 below). On the day of the surgery, after procedure, she stopped breathing. The doctors bagged and pumped her chest (performed CPR) until one mistake turned out to be a blessing. While replacing the trach tube, the doctor asked for a "2.0" (which is the length or size of the trach tube) and was given a "2.5" instead. It turned out the 2.0 that was originally inserted was too short. The 2.5 was perfect, and her breathing improved. Her numbers (stats) went up (i.e., oxygen saturation and heart rate). This was the first time my baby was able to breathe without struggling, and it was the first time I had seen her face without tape or tubes covering it. (Shown in photograph 3)

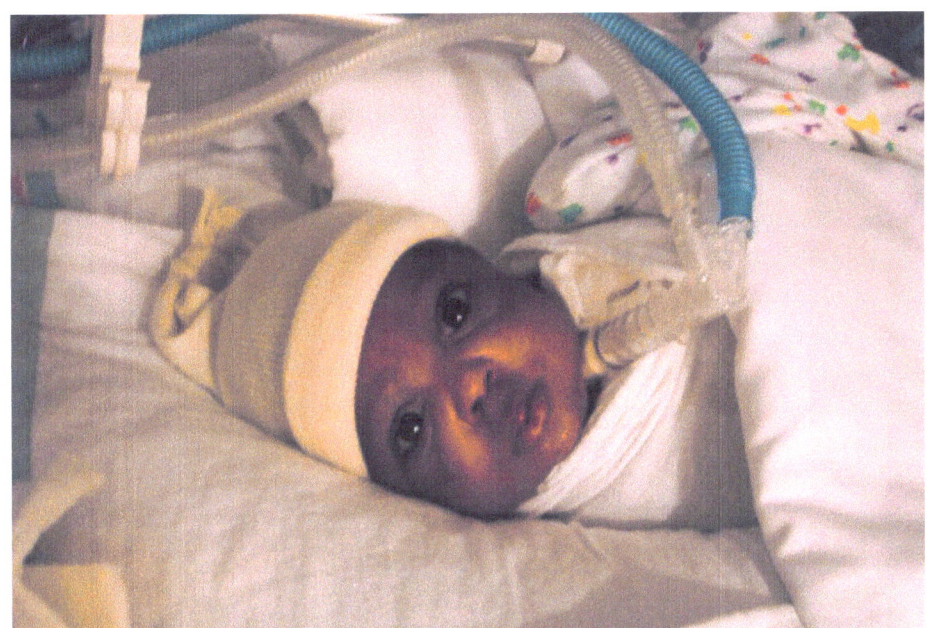

Photograph 3. Day of tracheotomy

I CAN SEE YOUR FACE

For the first time, Thea had no tapes, wires or CPAP tubing blocking her face. Her first smile was my greatest present.

She was five months and two weeks old when the decision to go to rehab was discussed, in order to prepare us to take her home. We had to choose between two hospitals: one which was close to our home or one out of state. A nurse advised me to pay attention to the infection rate, the sanitation, and the respiratory care/staff, etc. It is always a good idea to ask questions and have a good relationship with the nurses and doctors taking care of your child. You might be surprised how much you can learn from them, such as tips or information that they would not normally tell you otherwise. I took all the information I gathered, and we made the decision and chose the rehabilitation hospital upstate in Westchester.

Making the choice was the easy part. Getting in was another story because the rehabilitation hospital was ranked as the best for respiratory care—the space was limited.

This is where the relationship you have with the staff at the hospital is going to count, as top doctors collaborate with other top doctors, nurses with other nurses, and social workers with other social workers from other hospitals.

CHAPTER 2

Moving to Rehabilitation Hospital

ROAD TRIP TO REHAB

Thea was transported to Westchester by ambulance because she was on ventilation support. The ambulance was on time, but it was not equipped to carry an infant on respiratory support. Another ambulance was dispatched, which was better equipped to make the journey with an infant. It was amazing to see most of the hospital staff had come by to say goodbye to Thea: the maintenance staff, the NICU staff, the kitchen staff, the respiratory department staff and the PICU staff. I never knew one little girl's will to live would touch so many people.

COPING WITH RELOCATING TO REHAB

Again, new doctors, social workers, respiratory therapists, speech therapists, occupational therapists, and physical therapists—all in one day. I did not understand why a five-month-old needed a speech therapist and all the other therapists if we were there for breathing issues. It was explained that an early intervention is required to help her to catch up physically (because she was a premature baby with medical issues), and she would need help through the different stages of her development.

It was important to ensure that Thea settled into her new surroundings by keeping things as familiar as possible using crib toys, pictures, and any toys she (became accustomed to) had in PICU at previous hospital.

Since this is the last step in the road to going home, you should start to think about how his or her room would be decorated (look), when you get home. You should put a few of those things around for her to get use to them.

In most rehabilitation hospitals, the cribs can appear very cold and look like steel animal cages. Check with the hospital staff for permission to dress up the crib with a comfortable crib sheet set or crib bumper (shown in photograph 4 and 5). The purpose for this is to prepare your child for a smooth transition when they go home.

You should also start getting your child into a routine such as reading to him or her at a certain time of day (before naptime and before bedtime at night). If the rehabilitation center has rocking chairs, utilize them. Request to have one placed at your bed side, the rocking motion can be very soothing and comforting. You might also want to invest in one for home, because your child will get used to having story time while being rocked, and this will be a lifesaver once you get home.

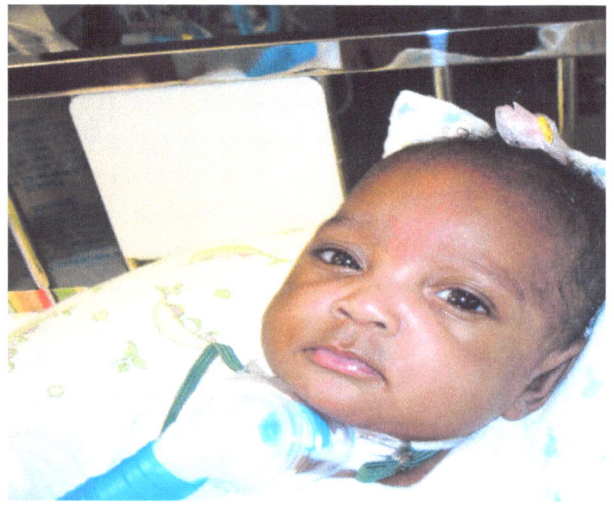

Photograph 4. Crib before crib sheet and bumper were added

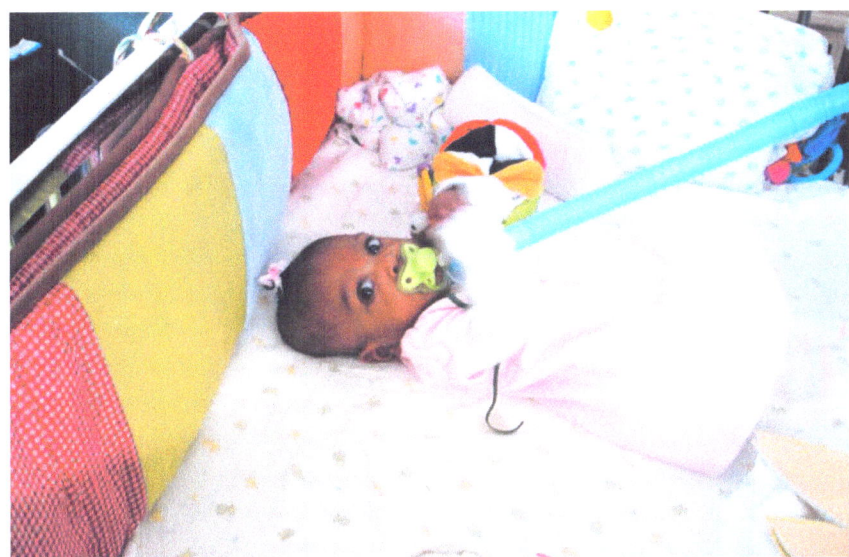

Photograph 5. Crib after crib sheet and bumper were added

Try to do your child's laundry yourself. This will prevent infection or skin irritation and lost clothing. This will also help you prepare for going home.

When it is medication time, as long as it is not an injection, ask the nurse to allow you to give it to your child. This will help you to practice and make it easier for you to administer once you go home (your child would be accustomed to you giving the medication). Always double check the dose with the nurse even though it is prepared (measured) by the nurse, this will help you to get familiar with the dose as shown on the syringe.

It is very important to try and keep a detailed journal of your child's activity; this should include the following:

1. The time medication is given and the type of medication.

2. Time respiratory treatment is given and how much.

3. Who is your child's nurse (date and time of shift)?

4. How much your child eats (consumption)? This will give you an idea if your child is eating well or not.

5. Frequency of bowel movements. (this will alert you if your child is not passing stool as frequently as he or she should).

You might think this is a lot of work, and you do not have the time, just do your best. Plus, there would be times when you would be too worried to remember everything, and believe me, you cannot! Your journal will relieve some of your stress, especially when you get home; and if you are not sure about something, you can refer to your journal for help. In addition, make yourself familiar with your surroundings because that's where you will be for the next couple of months. You being there is all the security your child needs.

Most rehabilitation hospitals have parent housing, don't hesitate to ask if it is not offered. I was relieved when I was offered a place to sleep (parent housing) for the first two weeks. Then, it was on a week-by-week basis based on availability of rooms. At the end of each week, I would find my social worker and apply for another week. I did not have a problem with that because I was not going to leave Thea under any circumstance even if it meant sleeping in a chair at her bedside.

If possible, do not leave your child unattended for a long period of time at any hospital for several reasons listed below:

1. Hospital staffs are overworked and do not have time to sit and comfort your child (if he or she cries), because they have more than one patient assigned to them. They might be dealing with another patient and your child might have difficulty breathing, then you can alert someone.

2. Your job is to hold your child when he or she needs comforting and to cater to his or her every need. Basically, keep your child happy as this will help your child to concentrate on healing, not fussing. This will help their condition to improve.

3. In the event your child's trach tube slips out, or get disconnected from the respiratory machine, you will be there to summon help quickly. Keep in mind, a person can only go three to five minutes without oxygen, before serious damage is done to the brain. (In the event, tell yourself you only have three minutes, this way you work faster to reduce the chance of serious damage).

4. Your presence is important, remember you are your child's advocate.

5. Being there gives you the opportunity to learn faster and your child will be able to go home faster. Be vigilant; pay attention to the respiratory therapist. You must ask questions, that is how you learn and knowing will help you later if there is an emergency.

The best thing to do this is to make the sacrifice and stay with your child. You will get very exhausted, but you won't be happy otherwise, and you will have peace of mind. It is important to take a day off if you have a spouse or grandparent who is willing to take over for a day or two. Remember you are no help to your child if you are exhausted. This is where family support is important.

After six weeks at the rehabilitation hospital, we were told that Thea could go home. This was due to the fact that I had been a hands-on-parent; I paid attention, and I learned fast. However, they had to be absolutely sure we could cope at home. There were series of tests we had to take: to prove we could operate the respirator correctly, to be able to give her treatment using the nebulizer correctly, and to take a CPR class (at least two family members had to be trained).

One week after we completed all the requirements, and all departments gave us a passing grade, we were given the biggest test of all. We were allowed to take Thea home for the weekend as a test run. We had to check her back into the rehabilitation center by the following Monday before noon.

We were equipped with portable ventilator with tubings, oxygen tank, and pulse oxamiator (which monitor her heart rate and oxygen levels), suction pump, suction catheter, respirator, and extra trachea tubings (in case the one she had in got blocked). We had everything needed to care for her for the weekend.

The weekend was exciting and scary at the same time. We were happy she was finally home, but I had to remind myself we had to take her back. The look on her little face as she took in her new surroundings was priceless. It was as if she knew this was home. We sat in her rocking chair and we began story-time. She was comfortable because this had become our little routine (mommy–and–me-time), and she quickly fell asleep. She was placed in her crib for her first nap at home.

On Monday, we loaded up and got ready for the long, two-hour ride to Valhalla. When I got out of the car in front of the hospital, I was relieved. We did it; we got through our weekend without any problems. I was ready. The hospital had to put a few things in place now that the test run home was successful. Certain preparations had to be made: medical supply company, nursing, and occupational therapy (OT), physical therapy (PT), and speech therapy had to be established.

A representative from the medical supply company came to speak with us, and made arrangements to drop off machines, and made sure we knew how to use them. Once the nursing was finalized, we were free to go home. We stayed at the rehabilitation hospital for a total of two months.

CHAPTER 3

Going Home

FINALLY GOING HOME

Every parent dream of bringing home their baby, but bringing home a critically ill child is one of the scariest times in any parent's life. Being prepared for it is even more important. This is the test of all tests where parents put everything they have learn to use. Do not worry because you have been taking care of your child all along, preparing you for coming home, and homecare. If you survive the first week, then the next week will be easier, and before you know it, one week will turn into one month, and a month will turn into a year.

My first night home did not go as smooth as my weekend. It was the longest night of my life because the air compressor the medical supply company delivered was not as quiet as the one we had for the weekend from the rehab hospital. I could not hear if Thea was having difficulty breathing, so I had to stay awake the entire night, and watch her breathe, because it was very noisy. The next morning, I called the medical supply company and told them to send someone to check the compressor because it was noisy. When the representative of the supply company arrived, I explained the problem to him. He informed me there was a quieter model. He was surprised that I was given that one in the first place. He telephoned the company, and requested the quieter model, and he waited for it to arrive.

Helpful Tips for Tracheostomy Care

As a parent and the caregiver of your child, keep in mind that if you are not happy with anything from the medical supplier, do not hesitate to call and request something different, or ask for suggestions from your contact person at the company (person assigned to your account). Make sure you have a good relationship with them because you have to work as a team, and if all goes well you will be working together for years as long as everyone is on the same page.

The following are points to keep in mind when dealing with a medical supply company:

1. It is best to write or type your list and fax it to that person; make sure you write model numbers, manufacturer, size, and color, if possible. Be specific to avoid any mix-up. All of the information can be found on packaging you use from the hospital. If the medical suppliers do not have the particular brand you want, and you have a good relationship with the person assigned to your account, they will go the extra mile to try and get it.

2. Always make sure you keep a folder with any information you fax and delivery receipts for your records; and check to make sure you have received what you have signed for.

3. Always make sure you have at least two tracheotomy tubes in stock (the size you use and size down in case of swelling of tracheotomy site) which does not include the one in your child's neck.

4. Try not to wait until you are low or out of supplies to order. By now, you should know what you need, and how fast the supplies are used.

5. Know the quantity your insurance pay for per month (the medical supply company have this information), this will help you to stretch your supplies so you will not run out before the month is over; this will also help to reduce out off pocket cost.

CHOOSING THE RIGHT NURSES

Choosing the right nurse can be complicated. However, this is based on your child's condition and the amount of hours given by your insurance provider.

Make sure the company sends qualified nurses based on your child's needs and make sure they meet the qualification the insurance company is paying for. If your insurance company is paying for a registered nurse, the identification on name tag should read registered nurse (RN) and not license practical nurse (LPN). This can be a stressful time; hence, you want to make sure that your nurse is capable of performing his or her duties and backing you up if there is a problem. You do not want someone to freeze on you when your child's life is at stake. In addition, make sure the company has a full understanding of your child's medical condition and that they inform the nurses that are sent to you. I had a situation with one of the nurses sent to my home. She was shocked to see that my child had a tracheotomy because she was told she had another illness and was hooked up to a respirator. To avoid this situation, it is important to interview them when they arrive. This should be done before introducing them to your child.

I decided to reduce the number of nurses that frequent my home to three. Since I would train them how to care for my child, and as soon as I was comfortable to trust them to care for her, the agency would send a new nurse. I found myself retraining a new nurse every few days. As a result, I changed my strategy and put the following plan below into motion, which I think worked very well:

1. Ask if they have ever worked with a patient with tracheotomy, what they did if possible, and for the steps in caring for a patient with tracheotomy.

2. Have the nurses demonstrate how to suction. This way, you would know if they have ever suctioned a person before. This will save you a lot of headache and make your choices simple. (The last thing you want to do is leave your child with someone who doesn't

know what they are doing.)

3. If you decide to keep the nurses, teach them how you want them to suction your child (how far they should go with the suction catheter), this depends on the size of the tracheotomy tube (see photograph 10, 11, and 12 on page 31).

4. Introduce your child to the nurse and pay close attention to the way your child responds to the nurse. By now, you should know your child and how he or she reacts to people. Trust your child because they are the one who will be dealing with the nurse and also trust yourself.

    There was this one nurse that my daughter smiled and reached out to the moment she walked in. I had to keep that nurse as they were great together (I trained her to care for my child). She would smile at other nurses, but would not go to them or let them touch her. This is not good because you want your child to be comfortable with whomever you leave her with, and peace of mind for you as well.

5. You should limit your nursing staff to three to eliminate the agency from sending you a new nurse every few days. This will help you to cut down on the amount of traffic that frequents your home. You can also keep the risk of infection under control. Allow at least two weeks before limiting your staff to three, that way they would have sent enough nurses for you to hand pick the three you want.

6. Because of your child's breathing condition, make sure the nurses you choose do not smoke. I had one nurse that showed up to work after she had a cigarette. I asked her if she is a smoker. She told me (stated) she does not, but her boyfriend smokes. I told her sorry; but I could not use her, and she had to go because of my child's respiratory condition. I called the agency and informed them of the situation to prevent that from happening again.

7. Be sure to check identification when you meet the nurses for the first time, to ensure that they are who they say they are, and have the appropriate qualification.

8. During the interview with nurses, explain your house rules and any other concerns you may have.

9. If possible, always have two people with your child at all times in case of any emergency. One person would be able to dial 911; while the other concentrates on saving your child. In addition, if one person freezes, the other person will jump into action.

10. During interviews, please instruct your nurses to change into scrubs at your home (when they get to work). Do not wear the scrubs on public transportation or on the street (remember you are trying to keep infection under control).

CHOOSING THE RIGHT THERAPIST

Early intervention plays a very important role in your child's life; not only because he/she is a premature baby, but because of his or her illness. Your child might be delayed with eating or chewing issues, speech or physical impairments. In Thea's case, she had a little of everything:

1. Very weak upper and lower body strength because she had to lie down for all those months (first few months of her life) because she was attached to one machine after the other.

2. She also had sensitivity issues with her hands because as a premature baby, she was constantly poked with needles for one test or the other, and because she had numerous surgeries as well.

3. She had problems chewing solid food without gagging on it.

It is very important to know who your case worker (social worker) is. Have a good relationship with her or him, as this is the person you will be working with (for the first three years of your child's life) if there is a problem with your therapist and you wish to change your therapist or if you wish to increase or decrease your child's sessions.

Choosing the right therapist can be difficult. We went through several speech therapists before we found the right one. One therapist refused to wash her hands when she entered my home even after I explained how important it is to prevent infection to my child. Another therapist had no patients and should not have been working with children. Thea refused to go to few therapists so they were dismissed after several wasted sessions.

Not only do you want good therapists, but you want therapists that are reliable and show up when they are scheduled; and not whenever they feel like it, as this will cause them to overlap with another therapist.

When having therapists to work with your child, you should:

1. Therapist credentials should be checked the same as your nurses, explain your infection concerns and let them know your house rules. Use this time to tell them that if they are sick or think they are catching a cold to call and cancel their session. Under no circumstances, contact with your child should not be allowed if the therapist is sick because of your child's weak immune system.

2. Again, anyone entering your home should wash their hands with soap and water before using hand sanitizer. Most people think, by using sanitizer, their hands are clean. Studies show that after using hand sanitizer a few times, you should wash with soap because the

hand sanitizer becomes ineffective.

3. If possible, clean gowns should be provided by you, and placed at the entrance to your home (shown in photograph 6). These should be worn after they wash their hands before contact with your child to prevent or cut down on cross-contamination (infection). Keep in mind, therapists have more than one client and you are not always the first one they see that day.

4. Make sure your child responds to the therapists, in that way, she will look forward to having therapy with them, and not cry or get unhappy whenever they walk in. This does not mean your child will want to have therapy all the time, but what we are hoping for is most of the time.

5. Make sure the therapists show up when they are scheduled to, and not before or after their session. This can cause therapy sessions to overlap. They are not to go over into the other therapist's time if they are late. They should stop at once or at least half an hour before the other therapist arrives.

6. Under no circumstances should you allow one session after another (back to back). This will tire your child and can be very overwhelming to your child. One session should be done in the morning and the other in the afternoon or after naptime, this will give your child time to rest between sessions.

7. Therapists are allowed to work out their schedule (switch sessions) with each other but the final changes should be approved by you at least a week in advance.

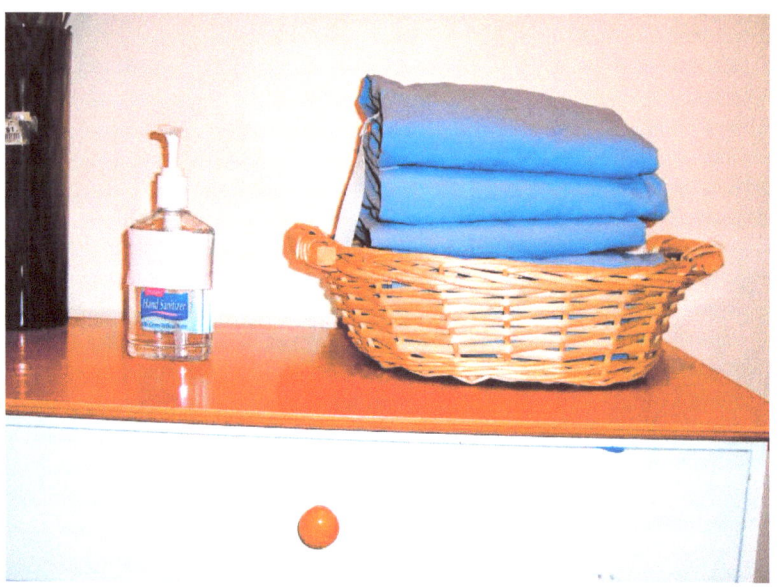

Photograph 6. Clean gowns

Every three months, your child will be given a progress report to assess if your child is meeting his or her goals or not. Your child's therapy hours might be decreased or increased. If they are decreasing the hours, and you do not think your child is meeting his or her goals, you can request for the hours to remain the same, or increase if necessary. Here again is where your case worker will assist you in the process. Never hesitate to speak up if you think your child needs more hours or a different therapist because you are your child's advocate. You have to make sure he or she gets what is best for him or her.

On your child's third birthday, he or she will "age out" of early intervention. Your social worker or caseworker should help you set up a meeting with the Committee on Preschool Special Education (CPSE), for your child to be issued a new therapist. You will be assigned a new caseworker who will assist you with finding new therapist. Your child will also be assigned a teacher (SEIT) base on your child's medical condition that teacher will come to your home.

Do not be surprised if you are given a phonebook-sized contact list of therapist (OT, PT and SP) numbers to assist in finding a therapist for your child, this is not an easy task and it can be overwhelming.

CHAPTER 4

Tracheotomy Care

TRACH TIME

It is always best to do trach time after a bath, so your child can associate it with bath time. Always try to carry out trach time in the same location so your child knows what time it is and how to behave when he or she is in that position or location. Parent or caregiver should always suction child before trach care to insure airway is clear.

Don't be afraid to play a little with your child (funny faces are fun), before and during trach time. This lightens the mood and get him ready for your little demonstration. Most importantly, after every trach change, let your child know how much you appreciate him keeping still and helping you during trach time. you can kiss him or hug him based on the medical condition of your child. If your child is active, give them both, and if they are not active, give extra kisses.

Always check to make sure trach collar is not too tight or too loose and is clear of anything that can cause your child to reach back, and unfasten the tie (this can be hair or label in your child's clothing), (see photograph 7 below). The last thing you want is for your child to realize he or she can release the collar and take the tracheotomy tube out, this can be very dangerous.

Helpful Tips for Tracheostomy Care

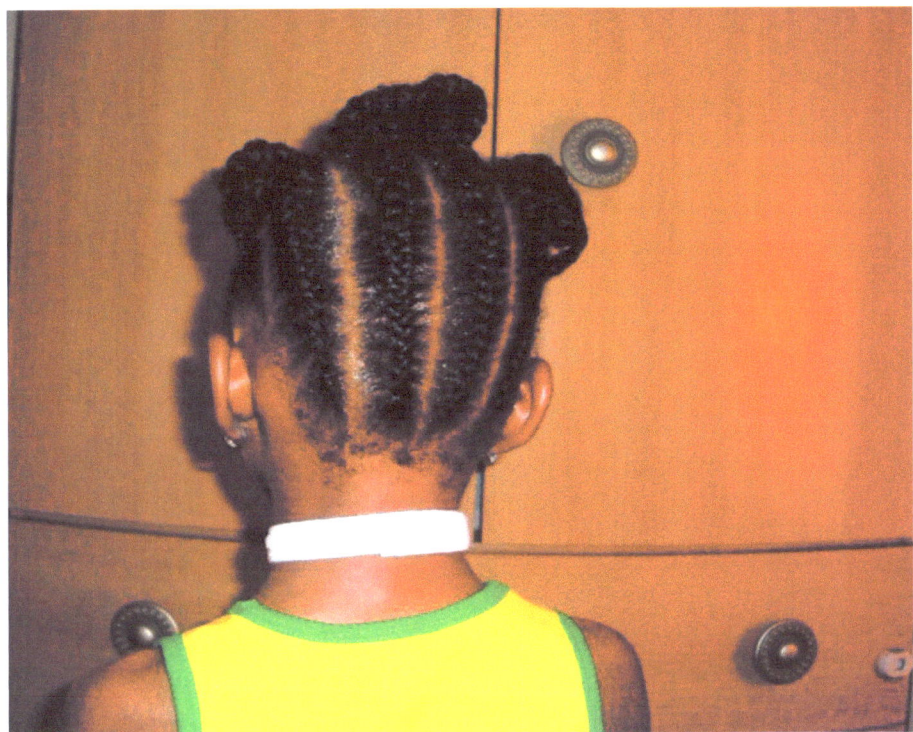

Photograph 7. Back of the neck without hair or clothing label

Most important in case of an emergency, have an emergency kit (see photograph 8) which is easily accessible to you or anyone caring for your child next to the area where trach time is done, or area where your child spends most of his or her time (always keep trach supplies out of a child's reach). This kit should include:

1. Tracheotomy collar (trach collar).

2. Trach tube (in case the tube gets clog, and you have to change it in a hurry, it would be easily accessible to you)

3. Drain sponge (non-woven IV dressing sponges) are best to prevent thread from getting into trach site; they are very easy to maneuver because they are precut. (Shown in photo 8)

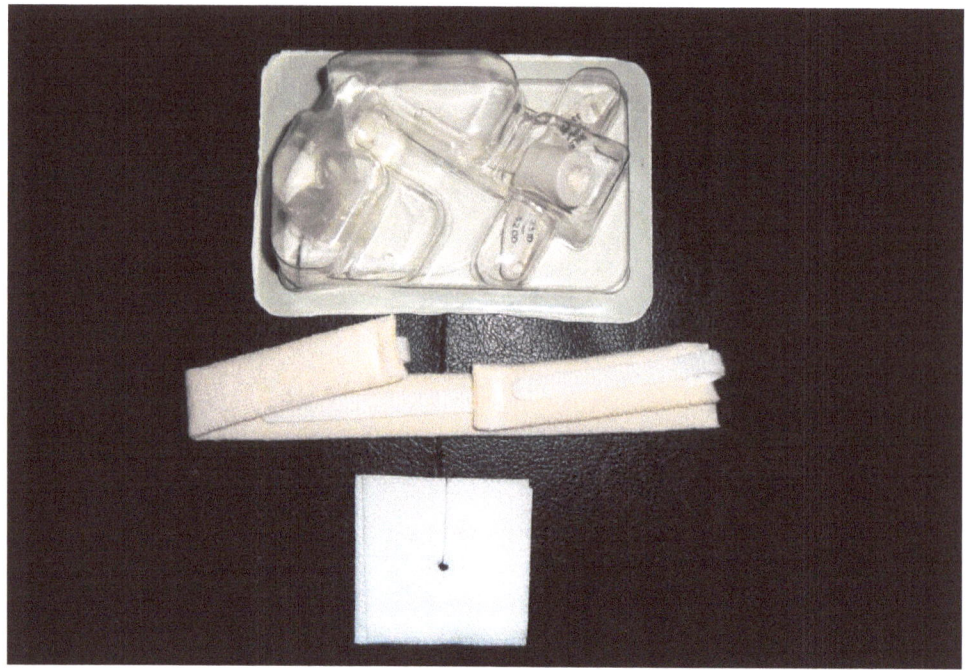

Photograph 8. Trach tube, collar, and drain sponge

PREPARING SUPPLIES FOR TRACH MAINTENANCE OR TRACH TUBE CHANGE

While preparing the trach supplies, be sure to get your child involved (no matter what's the age of the child), explain the steps of what you are doing. This little demo will help them feel comfortable about trach time and become accustom to having their trach cleaned or changed (it can also be used as dad-and-me or mom-and-me time). It is so amazing how fast a child learns, just by watching you, and listening to you talk. It also distracts them from wanting to move or play with their toys. Hold everything up to your child's eye level, so they can see what you are doing. Act like you are enjoying it, so they will enjoy watching you, and enjoy trach time (remember if you are not happy, they are not happy).

1. Mom/dad is preparing cleaning solution. (let your child see what you are doing as you say it)

2. Mom/dad is cutting trach collar. (cut tie to child's neck size for comfort)

3. Mom/dad is getting cotton. (if cotton balls are large, cut them in two to save cost)

4. Mom/dad gets drain sponge (in some cases to save cost, it is easier to purchase 4x4 and cut them into 2x2; this will give you four). Be sure to cut a line down the middle and create a hole for the trach tube, this gets easier with practice. (Shown in photo 9)

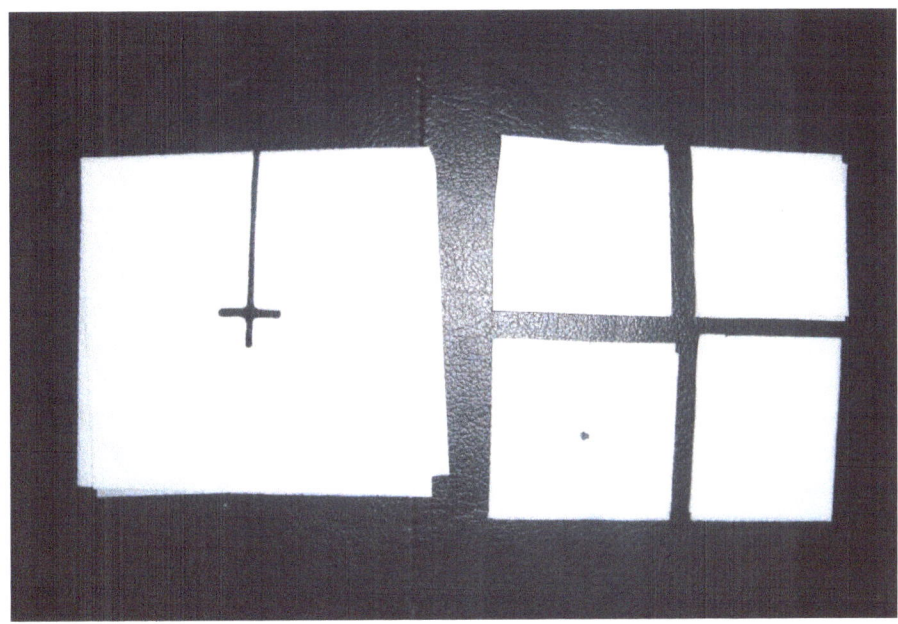

Photograph 9. Drain sponge

Drain sponge is very important because it helps to prevent excess drainage from the trach site, and also prevents the trach site from getting a rash or infected. Often, if the drain sponge is not in place every time your child coughs, it leaks secretion around the sides causing the area to be wet. Eventually, you will get an odor from the site which would cause your child to itch around the area or pull at the tracheotomy tube. It is important that you keep the trach collar, drain sponge, trach tube, and area around neck clean at all times so you can tell if something is wrong or if it is starting to get infected. One sign that something is wrong is a foul smell from sponge indicating an infection. Do not hesitate to call your pediatrician or go to the emergency room. *Do not ignore it!* Remember to trust your instinct.

1. Always smell drain sponge (every time you clean) for odor; this odor is not the normal saliva smell you will know when you smell it. If this should occur, go to your pediatrician or emergency room (notify them of your concerns), and request to have the tracheotomy site tested (a culture). This test is not painful, all they are going to do is suction your child and test the secretion for infection.

2. Inspect drain sponge for discolorations; this can be yellow or mocha colored, also followed by an odor. **DO NOT IGNORE IT!** Call your pediatrician or go to the emergency room. Remember trust your instinct. It is always best if the doctor tells you that it is nothing than to do nothing ("Prevention is better than the cure").

SUCTIONING

Suctioning can be very intimidating at first for some people, you might think you are hurting your child, keep in mind you are actually helping them, which is why you should do your homework first.

It is very important to know your child's tracheotomy tube size and the size of suction catheter it uses. This will allow you to know how far you can go when you suction.

Helpful Tips for Tracheostomy Care

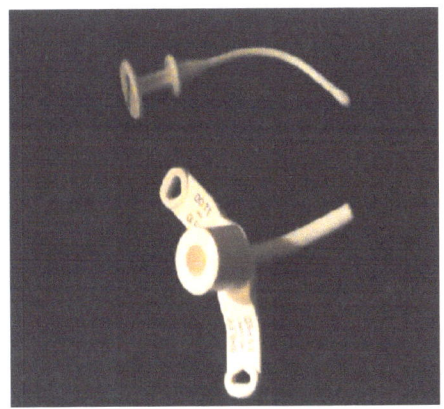

Photograph 10. Trach tube

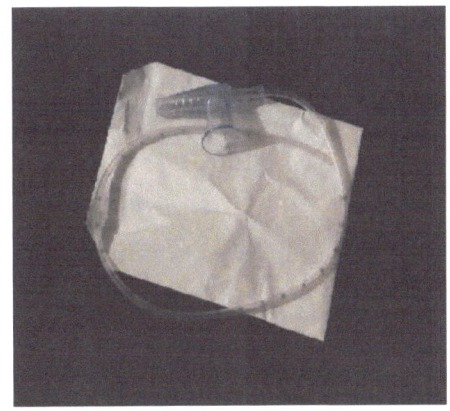

Photograph 11. Suction catheter

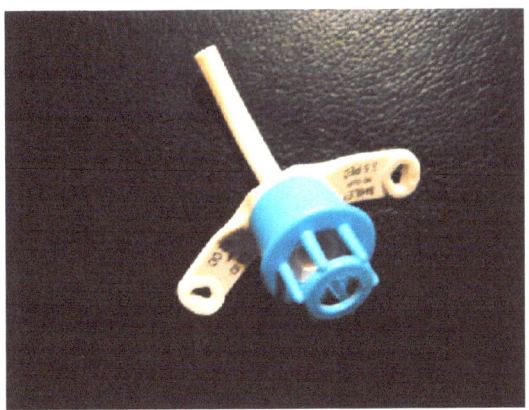

Photograph 12. Trach tube with extension

By measuring the length of the trach tube (an easy way to do this is by using an old trach tube and insert the suction catheter to see how far you can go before it sticks out of the bottom of the trach tube), you will have an idea how far you can go. Most suction catheters have numbers on them (from 4-26). For example, for a 3.5 pediatric trach, you would hold the suction catheter at the number six (6) if the child is wearing an extender, then you would hold the suction catheter at number eight (8). Make sure that you do not go too far beyond tracheotomy tube because this can cause scaring or other serious damage. Other signs that you have gone too far are:

1. Blood in the suction catheter or in secretion when your child or patient coughs after being suctioned is an indication you went too far.

2. Another sign is your child would gag when you suction him or her.

Most importantly, the person who will be suctioning your child must always make sure to wear gloves provided in the suction kit. If you are right-handed, use your left hand (if you are left-handed, use your right hand). This should be your sterile hand, because it is the hand you use least, this will take practice and some getting used to, but it will get easier.

INFECTION CONTROL

This is not an easy task, but the good news is it can be done by creating a system. Always keep in mind; say it to yourself, "I do not want to go back to the hospital except for checkups". In some cases, if you have a large family, this can be difficult to control especially if you have other children (of school age), or heavy traffic coming in (nurses, family members, friends and therapist) to your home. Everyone in your household and visitors need to work together as a team; in some instances you may have to put your foot down. Make it clear to your friends and family what your house rules are, and if they care for you and your child, they will help. The six rules listed below will help you to stay on top of infection.

SIX IMPORTANT HOUSE RULES TO REDUCE INFECTION

1. Inform your visitors if they have a cold, or think they have one these: runny nose, cough, sneezing, and allergies. Please do not visit. Make sure your friends and family understand the seriousness of these rules.

2. No shoes in your home; no exception (you might be surprised how much germs a pair of shoes carries).

3. Everyone that enters your home must wash their hands (no exceptions). Hands are the leading carrier of the cold and flu viruses. If you have a child with a trach or respiratory

issues, a cold would be the last thing you want your child to catch. A simple cold would mean readmission to the hospital or death.

4. If you have nurses that come into your home, it is important that they do not wear scrubs to come to your home (on public transportation or street). Instruct them to change into scrubs at your home. This will help to minimize infection, public transportations are not always the cleanest places, and scrubs should not be worn on them.

5. If your child gets early intervention (Occupational Therapy, Physical Therapy and Speech Therapy), have the therapists cover their street clothes with gowns. This helps to reduce cross contamination from child-to-child because it serves as a barrier between the therapist's clothes and your child. Therapists usually have more than one child per day who requires their services and you don't know what the illnesses the other children may have or if they have a cold.

6. One room in your home should be designated the quarantine room. No matter how hard you try, someone in your household will get sick (catch a cold or the flu). The sick person should stay in that room until he or she feels better, and most important, stay away from your child and out of child's room or play area.

CHAPTER 5

Possible Side Effects of Tracheotomy

POSSIBLE SIDE EFFECTS OF HAVING TRACHEOTOMY

The tracheotomy tube is a foreign body and your body reacts to anything that does not belong in it. In Thea's case, a polyp grew above the trachea tube this was preventing her from breathing through her nose. This was discovered one morning while she was sitting on the bed playing. I noticed she was having difficulty breathing while making a wheezing sound. This was a sound I had never heard before and very quickly, it went from bad to worse; she stopped breathing completely. Quick thinking, I removed the trach tube and replaced it with a new one and she started breathing. All I could do was hug her real tight and cry my eyes out because I was alone when it happened. After inspecting the trach tube I had removed, I noticed it was completely blocked.

I told my mother and the nurses what happened and instructed them what to do in case they heard her wheezing, so they would be prepared. I also made up an emergency kit which consisted of a trachea tube, drainage sponge, and trachea tie. I stuck it on the wall next to the bed in case she stopped breathing again (shown in photograph 7).

When it happened again, I was not at home but my mother and the nurse were prepared to act when they heard the sound I had explained to them. Before it got critical, they changed the trachea tube.

I took her to the doctor (ear nose and throat), and informed him of my concerns. A camera was placed in her nostrils and the doctor discovered there was a polyp blocking the airway to the nose this was preventing her from breathing through her nose. This had to be surgically removed to prevent the breathing problems from happening again.

The first surgery to remove the polyp did not go well. It was too hard (the outside was as thick as the skin of a pumpkin) for the instruments. The doctor was unable to remove it. We had to wait another two weeks before the second attempt was made. This time they had stronger instruments and it was successful. The doctor thought by removing the polyp, Thea would have been able to be decannulated. Decannulation is when your child is able to have his or her tracheotomy tube removed. This is normally done when the doctor thinks your child's medical condition is better and he or she is able to breathe on their own without assistance. However, when we went for the post operation visit, we were informed she could not be decannulated. At first, I was crushed because I had made all these plans. We were going to do all the things she was not able to do because of her trachea. During the examination, the look on his face told me something was wrong. He stated that she had excessive scaring on her vocal cord because she was intubated. As a result, they were paralyzed on one side. I was happy because previously, I had been told that both vocal cords were paralyzed. One was a big improvement, but it delayed her being decannulated. We were referred to another doctor who would be able to remove the scar tissue in order for both vocal cords to move.

This led to a series of surgeries after the scar tissue was removed. She also had her airway reconstructed (a small piece of rib was removed and placed in her neck), and several surgeries before (a total of eleven surgeries). Based on your child's medical diagnosis, be prepared for him or her to have several surgeries to correct their condition. No parent gets used to seeing their child go through surgery; but keep in mind your child gets his or her strength from you, if you are not comfortable, he or she won't be comfortable. You might want to put a few pre-surgery routine in place such as:

PRESURGERY TIPS

1. Decide which parent is going to be the one to take the child into the operating room; this will help the child to relax.

2. Pick a song to sing to your child while he or she is being sedated (our song was *This Little Light of Mine*). This also will help to calm your child and after a while he or she will sing along.

3. Make sure you explain to your child that they would be going to the hospital for surgery. A few days before surgery and the day of surgery, explain a little bit about the procedure to your child to ensure that when he or she sees the hospital, they won't be surprised and scared. This will help them to relax before and during surgery.

4. If possible, ask the nurses or doctor to make sure once she is transferred to recovery and before she wakes up, to come and get you. You will be at his or her bedside so when your child wakes up, you are the first one he or she sees.

5. When you check in, ensure the nurses, doctors and anesthesiologist know what operation your child will be undergoing, so there is no mix up as to what type of procedure is to be done.

6. Suction your child yourself before surgery to make sure the airway is clear, and instruct the person who will be suctioning him or her (during surgery) what number to hold the suction catheter so they won't go too far when they suction during surgery.

As a parent, you must always pay attention to your child's every need; by doing so, you will be able to keep your child happy and from worrying about anything except breathing. Parents must always keep in mind that a happy baby (child) is easier on you and will help your child heal faster. Whatever makes you unhappy also makes your child unhappy. A child always knows what mood a parent is in, because they are learning and they learn by watching you.

SOME EXTRA TIPS THAT WORKED FOR ME

1. If your child cries, "Please!" try to comfort him or her. Excessive crying can cause an increase suctioning or clogging in the trach tube due to increase secretion. The same way a normal nose gets blocked when they cry, the same thing happens to the trach tube. (Your child breathes faster, causing the secretion to harden, quickly blocking the tracheotomy tube). In Thea's case, this happened (crying) during a therapy session, and the trach tube got blocked and she stopped breathing.

2. Try to keep the room your child (sleeps) spends most of his or her time as cool as possible. Not too hot, as this may require you to use an air condition unit (A/C) more frequently than normal. I find Thea's breathing was better when the room was cool. This will require you to dress your child in appropriate clothing to make sure they are not cold.

3. An easy way to know if your child is cold is by feeling his or her hands; if it is cold, they are cold.

4. If you notice, your child is throwing up (vomit) more of his or her food (two of every

three bottles) after every feeding, you should try to use a pacifier directly after feeding. This will cause your child to continue to suck, reducing gagging reflex and the food will stay down. Also, keep in mind this will cause your child to get attached to the pacifier; do not worry, the important goal is for your child to keep his or her food down to maintain weight and calorie intake. You can always wean him or her off of the pacifier once your child's condition improves.

5. Also make sure your child is not moving around too much after eating, and is in an up right position for at least 20-30 minutes before putting him or her too lie down.

6. Very important: if you notice your child is NOT eating, but only taking small sips of water, see an ENT doctor at once; this could be acid reflux (this is common in premature babies and babies with tracheotomy). This can be very stressful if you have an ill child who is also not eating. This happen with Thea, she was throwing up most of her food and eventually she stopped eating. This can be controlled with medication.

7. Keep your child's head elevated to keep airway open, and it also help with acid reflux; this may require you to place a device under the head of the mattress to elevate it or a proper head and neck support pillow.

8. Always think outside the box and put your self in their position. Do not doubt yourself; if they don't look comfortable, most of the time they are not. Trust your motherly instinct. If you think something is wrong, then it is. You know your child, and he or she is depending on you. Simple things such as removing a label from your child's clothing can give your child one less thing to worry about, moving around too much after eating can cause an upset stomach.

Helpful Tips for Tracheostomy Care

9. Rocking your child at story time helps to calm your child and help with development. Whatever it is, no matter how small, your child's only concern should be breathing and being happy, nothing else.

As a parent, what you want to ask yourself is, 'Can you make the sacrifice to do what ever it takes to help your child get better faster than the time predicted by the doctors?' In Thea's case, we were told she would have her trach until age seven (7). I was determine to do whatever I had to, including quitting my job to be a full-time caregiver for my child, I was diligent about keeping infection, and hospital visits to a minimum (except for checkups). With prayers dedication, trusting my instinct, training, family support, and team work (with therapist, nurses, and doctors). Thea's trach was removed at age three and a half.

The road to decannulation was not always easy, but every surgery, doctor's appointment and all the sacrifice made the outcome worth it. We are blessed to have a happy, healthy, beautiful five-year-old.

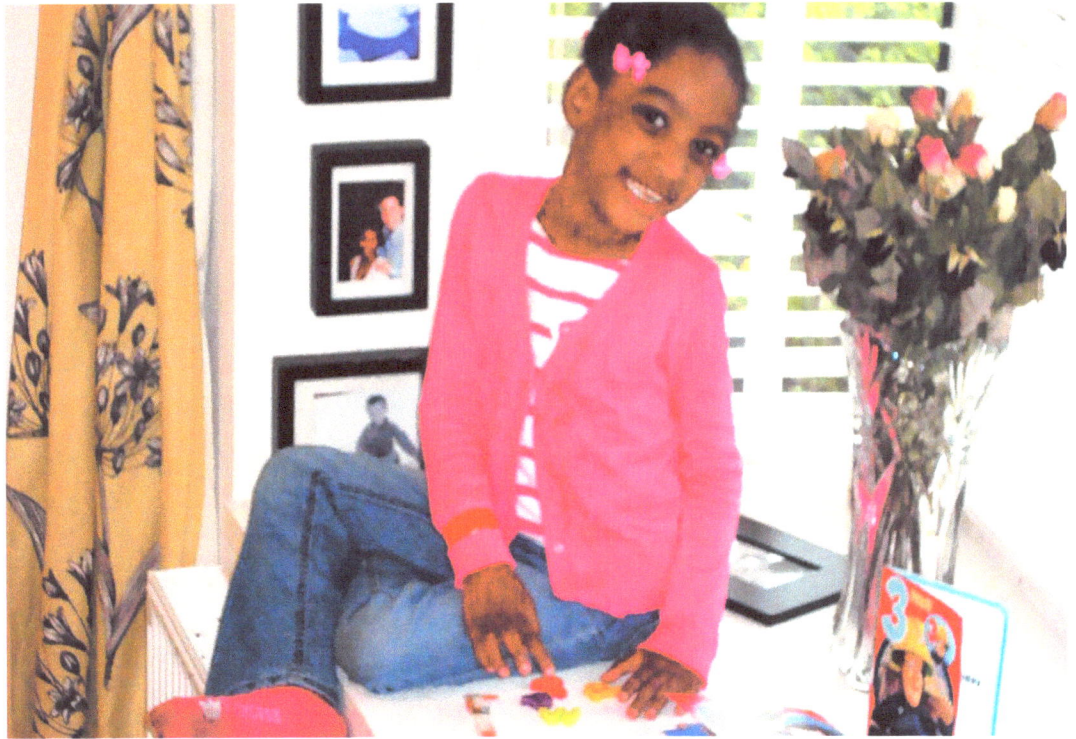

Photograph 13. Thea at age five

Sweet Reunion Pictures

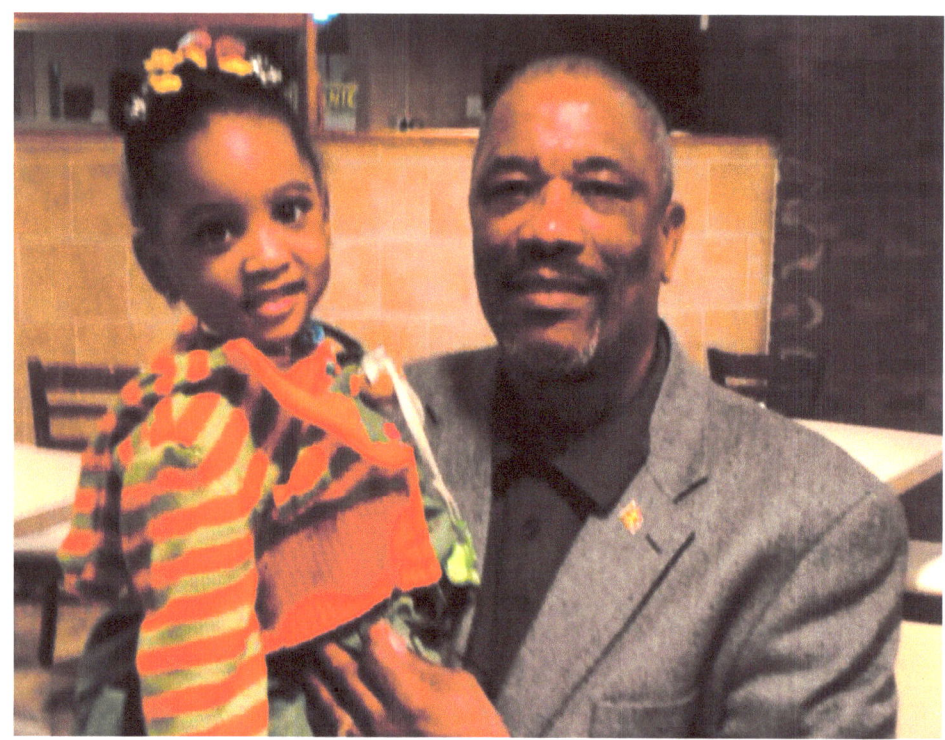

Photograph 14. Thea with respiratory therapist at hospital reunion

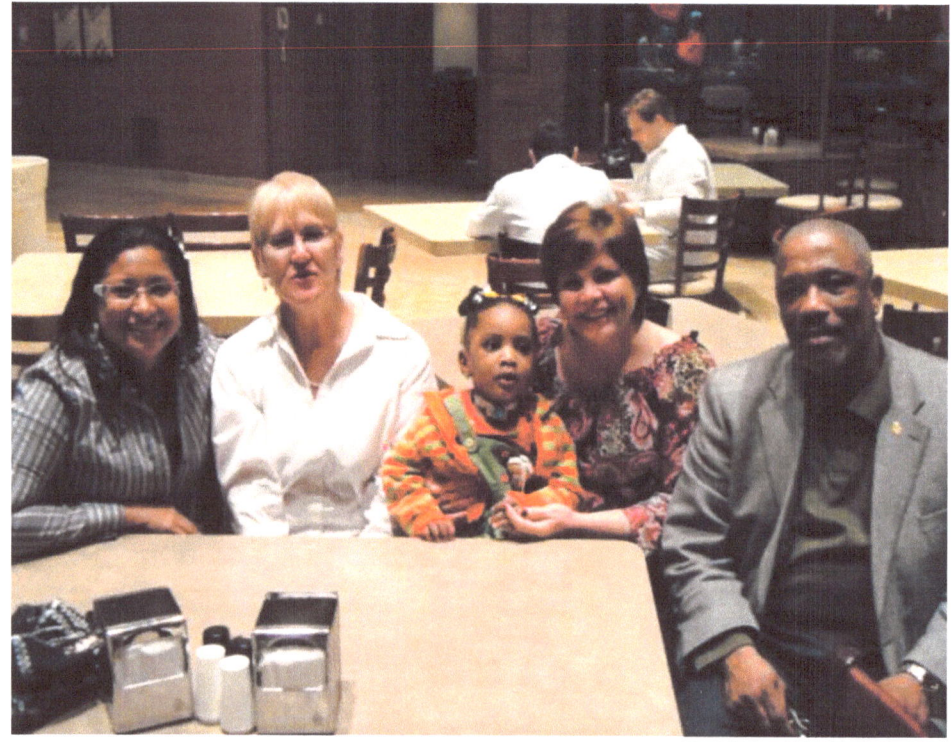

Photograph 16. Thea with NICU staff

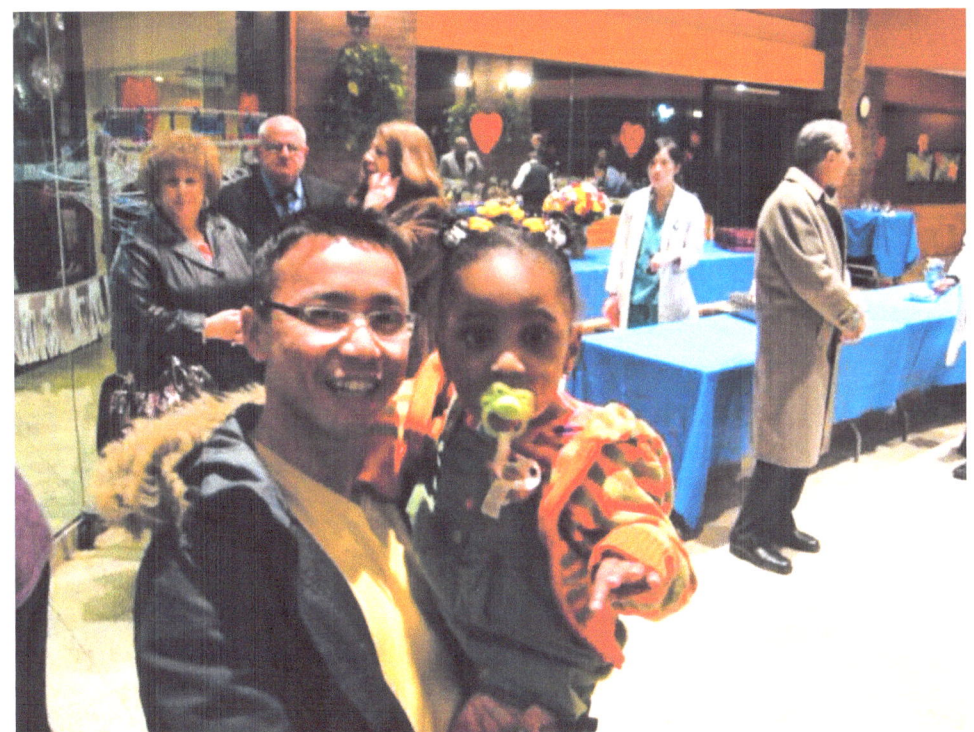

Photograph 17. Thea's pediatrician, Dr. Cao (www.southslopepediatrics.com)

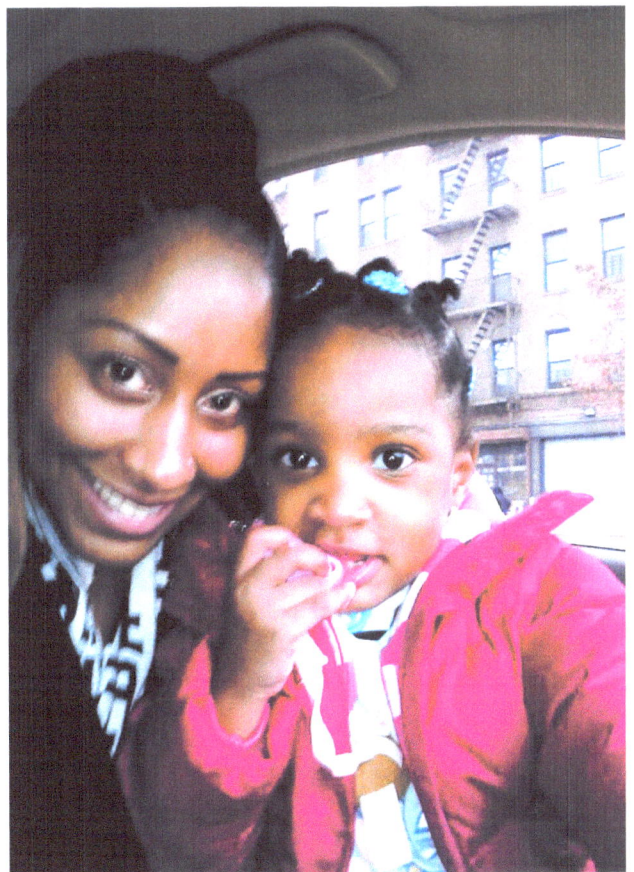

Photograph 18. Thea and Trinity, her nurse (thank you so much)

Index

A

acid reflux   38
age   28, 39
agency   19-20
airway   35-8
   insure   26
ambulance   11

B

baby   4-6, 8, 17, 37-8
   premature   11, 21, 38
breathe   4-5, 7-8, 17, 35
breathing   4, 8, 14, 17, 34-5, 37, 39
   started   34
breathing problems   35
breaths   4-5
   low-volume   5
brittle   4, 7
bumper   12-13

C

calm   36, 39
caregiver, full-time   39
case worker   22, 24
   new   24
chest, baby's   5
child breathes   37
child coughs   29
child cries   37
child-to-child   33
children   22, 32-3
child's activity   13
child's breathing condition   20
child's condition   19, 38
child's eye level   28
child's laundry   13
child's medical diagnosis   36
child's neck size   28
child's nurse   13
child's respiratory condition   20
child's tracheotomy tube size   30
clothing label   27
collar   26, 28
comfortable crib sheet set   12
comforting   5, 12, 15
company   17-19
   insurance   19
   medical   17
contact   22-3
contact person   18
contamination   33
Continuous Positive Airway Pressure (CPAP)   6-7
control   20-1, 32
Coretta Johnson   5-7, 9, 12, 16, 25, 28, 30-3, 35-7, 39, 41
cost   28-9
   pocket   18
CPAP (Continuous Positive Airway Pressure)   6-7
crib   12-13, 16
crib bumper   12
crib sheet   12-13
crib toys   12
cross-contamination   23

D

damage   15, 31
decision   8-9
   best   8
Diffusive Volumetric Respirator (DVR)   5-6
doctors   3-9, 30, 35-6, 39
   new   11
   pediatric   8
   top   10
doctor's appointment   39
dose   13
drain sponge   27-30
   smell   30
DVR (Diffusive Volumetric Respirator)   5-6

E

eating   14, 21, 38
Effects of Tracheotomy   34
emergency kit   27, 34
emergency room   29-30
ENT doctor   38

F

family 8, 32
  large 32
family members 15, 32
feeding 38
food 37-8
  solid 21

G

God 2
gowns, clean 23-4
grandparent 15

H

hair 26-7
hand sanitizer 22-3
hands 20-3, 32, 37
hands-on-parent 15
head 4, 6, 38
  child's 38
heart 2-3
heart rate 8, 16
home 9, 12-17, 19-24, 32-3, 35
homecare 17
homework 30
hospital 5-6, 9-10, 12, 14, 16, 18, 32-3, 36, 39
  rehab 17
hospital reunion 40
Hospital staffs 11-12, 14
Hospital Stay 4

hours 8, 19, 23-4
  child's therapy 24
household 32-3

I

identification 19, 21
infant 11
infection 13, 20-3, 29-30, 32-3
INFECTION CONTROL 32
infection rate 9
information 9, 18
instinct 29-30, 38-9
instruments 35
interviews 19, 21
IV dressing sponges, non-woven 27

J

journal 13-14

L

life 2-3, 6, 17, 21
  child's 19, 21-2
  parent's 17
life support system 6
location 26
lungs 4, 6-8
lungs time 8

M

machine 5-6, 15-16, 21
medical supply 16, 18
medication 13, 38
medication time 13
model, quieter 17
Mom/dad 28-9
Monday 16
Most rehabilitation hospitals 14
Most suction catheters 31
mother 2, 5, 34-5
  best 2
mother-in-law 2

N

neck 27, 29, 36
  child's 18
neck support pillow 38
NICU 4, 7
NICU doctors 7
NICU dreads 5
NICU staff 11, 40
noisy 17
nose 4, 34-5
  ear 35
  normal 37
  runny 32
nurses 3, 8-10, 13, 19-22, 32-6, 39, 41
  new 19-20
  qualified 19
  registered 19
  right 19
nursing staff 20

O

occupational therapists   11
occupational therapy (OT)   16, 25
odor   29-30
Oscillator   5-6
Oscillator and Diffusive Volumetric Respirator   5
OT (occupational therapy)   16, 25
oxygen levels   16
oxygen saturation   8
oxygen tank   16

P

pacifier   38
parent   3, 5, 7-8, 18, 26, 36-7, 39
parent dreams   17
parent housing   14
passing grade   16
patient   14, 19, 22
patient coughs   31
Pediatric Intensive Care Unit (PICU)   7-8, 12
pediatrician   29-30
person   15, 18-19, 21-2, 32, 37
person freezes   21
phonebook-sized contact list   25
photo   27, 29
photograph   5-9, 12-13, 20, 23-4, 26-9, 31, 34, 39-41
physical therapists   11
physical therapy (PT)   16, 25, 33
PICU (Pediatric Intensive Care Unit)   7-8, 12
PICU staff   11
polyp   34-5
premature child   5
pressure   6, 8
PT (physical therapy)   16, 25, 33

Q

qualification   19, 21

R

rehab   9, 11
rehabilitation hospital   10-12, 15-16
rehabilitation hospital upstate   9
relationship, good   9, 18, 22
relax   36
RELOCATING   11
respirator   15-16, 19
respiratory   15, 32
respiratory care   10
respiratory care/staff   9
respiratory department   6
respiratory department staff   11
respiratory distress   4
respiratory support   11
respiratory therapists   5-6, 8, 11, 15, 40
room   12, 14, 33, 37
    child's   33
    operating   36
quarantine   33
rules, house   21-2, 32

S

sacrifice   15, 39
scar tissue   35-6
scaring   31
    excessive   35
scrubs   21, 33
    wear   33
secretion   30-1, 37
    leaks   29
security   14
self   38-9
session   22-3
    switch   23
    wasted   22
shoes   32
sick person   33
sign   6, 29, 32
    bad   6
sing   36
soap   22
social workers   10-11, 14, 22, 24
song   36
sound   34-5
    wheezing   34
speech therapists   11, 22
speech therapy   16
staff
    kitchen   11
    maintenance   11
stats   6, 8
street clothes   33
strength, lower body   21

suction   19-20, 30, 32, 37
suction catheter   16, 20, 30-1, 37
suction child   26
suction kit   32
suction pump   16
suctioning   30, 32, 37
supplies   18
supply company   17
   medical   16-18
surgeries   8, 21, 35-7, 39

T

tapes   8-9
teacher   24
team   3, 8, 18, 32
   fresh   7
team work   39
test   15-17, 21, 30
Thea   3-6, 8-9, 11-12, 14-15, 17, 21-2, 34-5, 37, 39-41
Thea home   16
Thea's breathing   37
Thea's condition   5
Thea's miraculous improvement   6
Thea's pediatrician   41
Thea's trach   39
therapist credentials   22
therapists   3, 11, 22-5, 32-3, 39
   new   24
   right   21-2
therapist's clothes   33
therapist's time   23
therapy   23, 33
   occupational   16, 33
   physical   16, 33
therapy session   37
tie   26, 28
trach, pediatric   31
trach care   26
trach change   26
trach collar   27-9
trach color   26
trach site   27, 29
trach supplies   27-8
trach time   26-8
trach tube   8, 27-9, 31, 34, 37
   child's   15
trach tube photograph   31
trachea   4, 35
trachea tie   34
tracheotomy   8-9, 19, 34, 38
Tracheotomy Care   26
tracheotomy collar   27
tracheotomy site   18, 30
tracheotomy tube   18, 20, 26, 29, 31, 34-5, 37
transportations, public   21, 33
Trinity   3, 41
trust   19-20, 29-30, 38
tube   4-8, 27
   large   4
   trachea   34-5
tubings, extra trachea   16

U

use   6, 12, 16-18, 20, 22, 32, 37-8

V

ventilation   6
ventilation support   11
ventilator   5
   mechanical   4
   portable   16
visitors   32
vocal cords   35

W

wash   22-3, 32
weekend   16-17
weekend form   17
Westchester   9, 11
worry   17, 38

www.ingramcontent.com/pod-product-compliance
Lightning Source LLC
Chambersburg PA
CBHW051101180526
45172CB00002B/730